PENNY THE MEDICINE MAKER

We specialize in publishing quality books for
young people. For a complete list please write

LERNER PUBLICATIONS COMPANY

241 First Avenue North, Minneapolis, Minnesota 55401

PENNY
THE MEDICINE MAKER

The Story of Penicillin

By Sherrie S. Epstein

Illustrated by Mark Springer

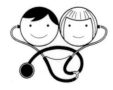

MEDICAL BOOKS FOR CHILDREN

LERNER PUBLICATIONS COMPANY
MINNEAPOLIS, MINNESOTA

International Standard Book Number: 0-8225-0006-X
Library of Congress Catalog Card Number: 60-14006

Eighth Printing 1973

Once upon a time, not so very long ago, there lived a good little germ. Like all germs, he was so tiny that he could only be seen through a microscope. This germ was named *Penicillium notatum,* or Penny for short, and this is the way he looked:

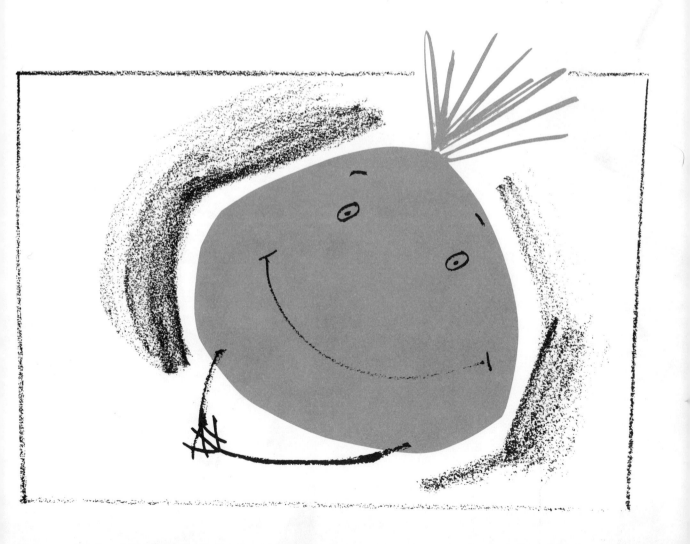

Not all germs are good. Some germs are bad because they make people sick. Some bad germs look like marbles. They are called "Staph" and are probably around when you get a pimple on your face. They look like this:

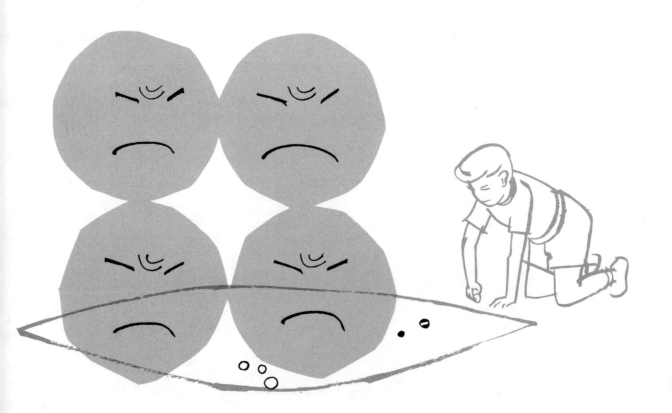

Some germs line up in rows like soldiers. They are called "Strep" and go out of the way to make your throat sore. Here is a chain of Strep:

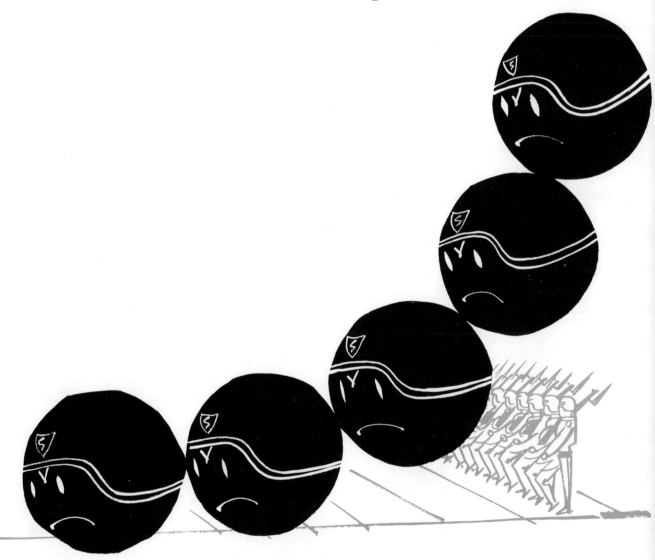

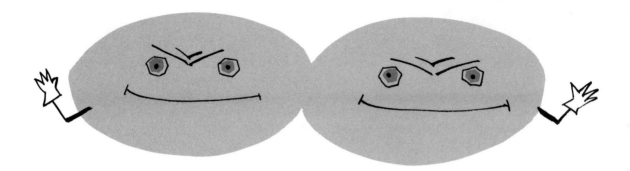

Other germs pair off like twin jelly beans. They are the "Pneumos" who are eager to make you cough and feel hot.

But Penny was not like any of these germs. He had a pleasant blue-green color. He was a shy fellow who spent most of his time taking a nap in a little boy's ear. It was warm and cozy there, and he heard thousands of television programs.

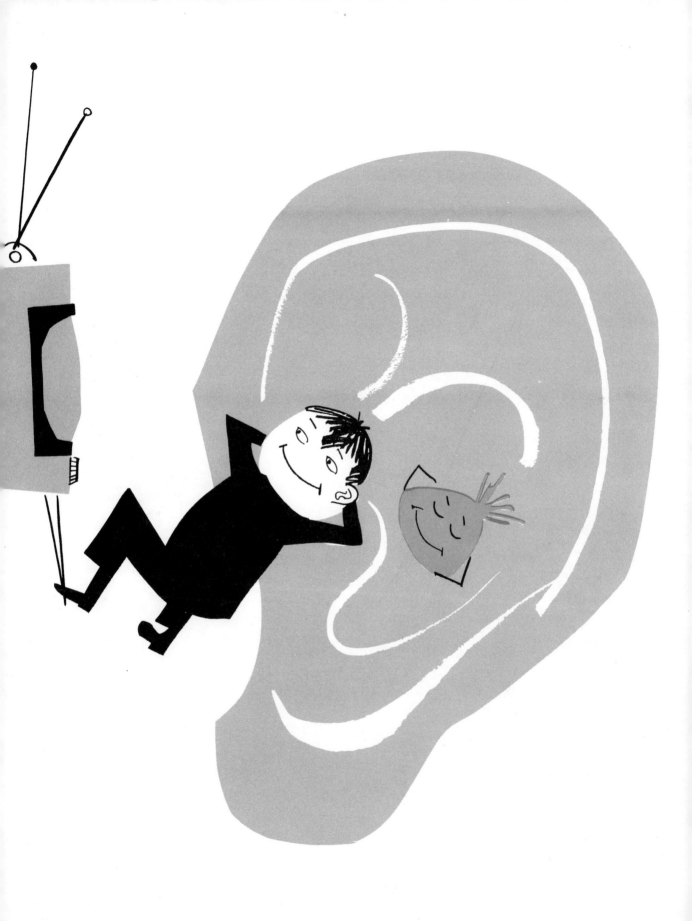

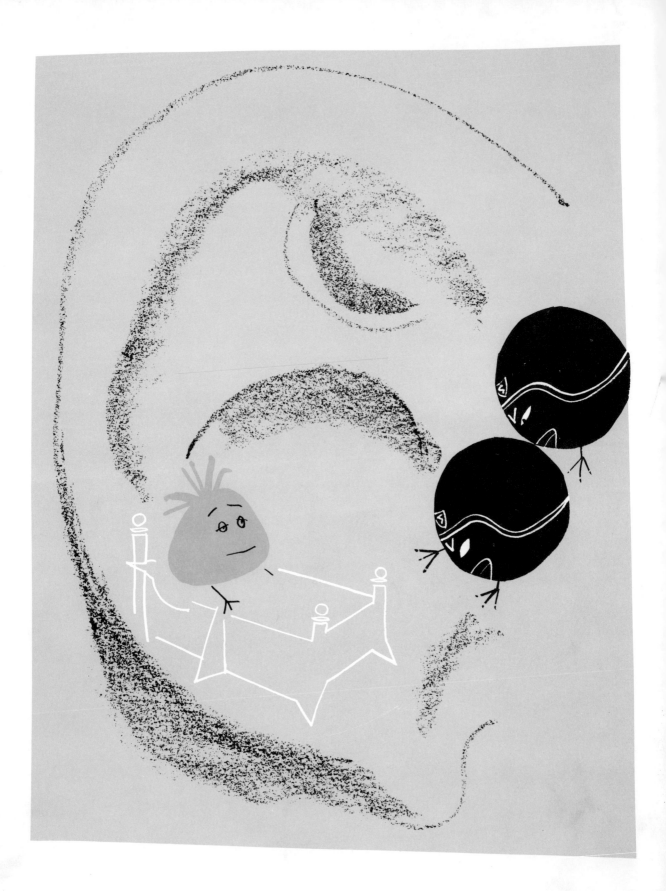

One day, Penny was awakened by a couple of strangers—small, round germs who looked rough and nasty. Penny gasped when he recognized them! They were Strep and they had a bad reputation.

Jumping up and down, the Strep hit and kicked the walls of Penny's soft, warm ear-house. "Come on, slowpoke," they called. "Didn't you ever learn how to ruin an ear?"

"No," Penny admitted. "What's the sense of doing that?"

"Sense-dense!" jeered the evil strep germs. "It's our job. If you're not going to help us, kindly leave!"

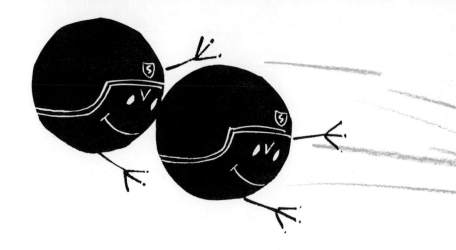

Before Penny could answer, they seized him and threw him out of the way. He tumbled down through the warm darkness until he bumped into the walls of the boy's throat. But there was no rest there! At least twenty more Strep were bouncing in and prancing around, grinding their teeth and screaming:

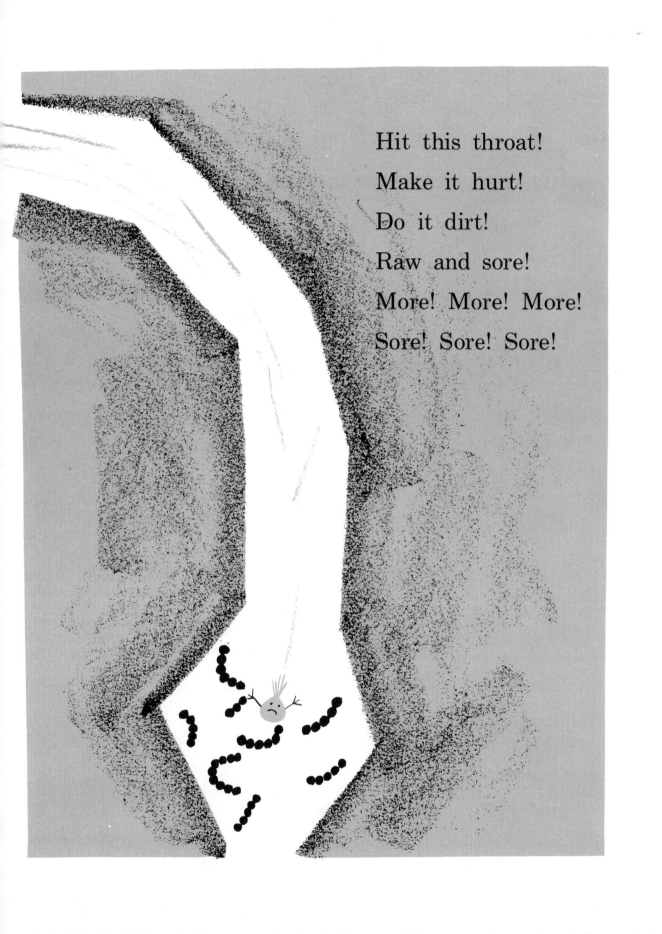

Hit this throat!
Make it hurt!
Do it dirt!
Raw and sore!
More! More! More!
Sore! Sore! Sore!

"No, no!" Penny shouted. "You're going to make this boy sick!" "Ho, ho!" laughed the Strep. "You catch on quickly, don't you!" Back they went to their war dance.

Just as they were singing their nasty song again, there was a loud noise. The little boy coughed and Penny found himself sailing out of the throat and floating through the air on a speck of dust. The wind blew him onto the leaf of a tree. Before he could catch his breath, the wind caught him up again and tossed him through the open window of a tall building.

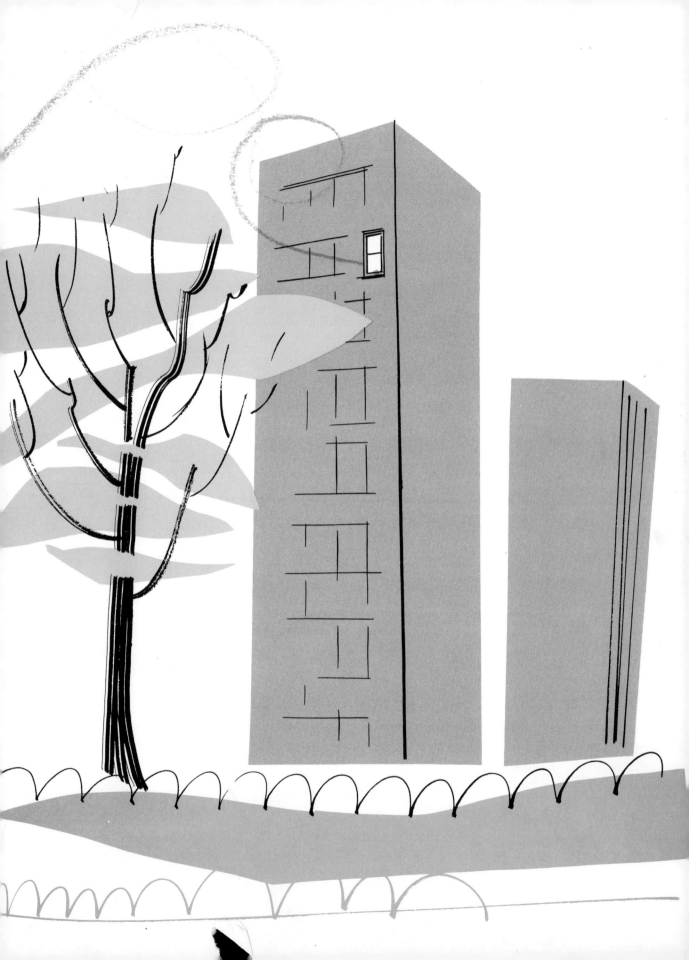

Plop!

Penny found himself in something soft and squishy that looked like lemon jello. He had landed in a dish on the table of a laboratory.

On the other side of the room, Penny could see a wise-looking man in a white coat. The man was Dr. Alexander Fleming and he was trying to grow different kinds of germs in other dishes just like the one in which Penny had landed.

Penny was angry! This dish wasn't as warm and pleasant as his old house in the boy's ear. Those Strep bullies had thrown him out of his home and had made a mess of it. Why, it might never be as comfortable again!

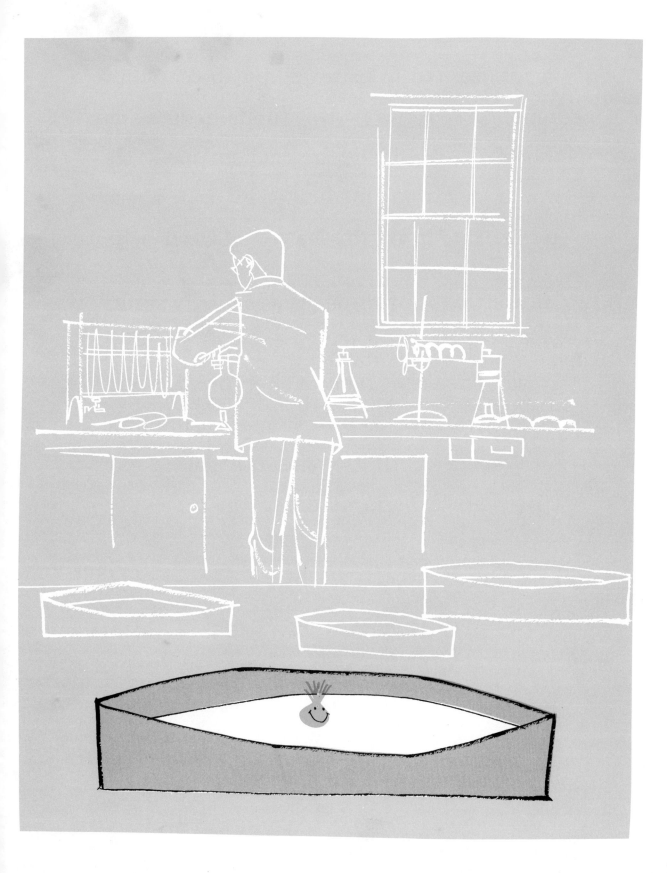

Penny wanted to get even, but he couldn't figure out a way. He thought and he thought, and finally he had an idea. He would make a medicine to kill those germs! But to do this he would need help.

He settled down on the squishy stuff and took a bite of it. He ate and ate, and grew. Then he took a big breath and pinched off a piece of himself. It didn't hurt a bit, of course, because germs like Penny are experts at doing this.

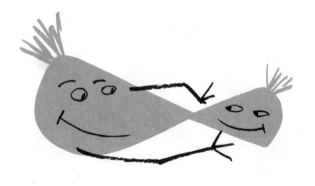

Where before there had been just one *Penicillium notatum,* now there were two! Each did the same thing over and over again until there was a whole angry tribe. There were so many of them that they could be seen even without a microscope. All of them together looked like a little tuft of blue-green fuzz.

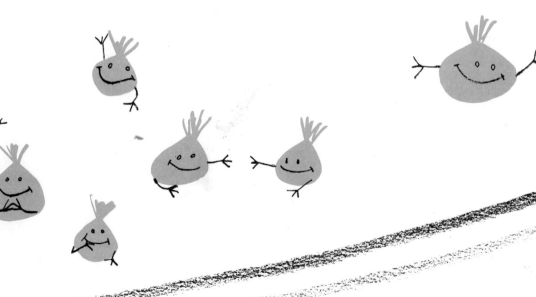

One at a time, each squeezed out a tiny drop of liquid that meant death to the Strep!

"Come on, gang!" Penny yelled. "Long live penicillin! Down with Strep!"

Just then, Penny heard Dr. Fleming's footsteps coming closer. "Dr. Alexander Fleming," Penny called; "here's some penicillin."

But Dr. Fleming just turned away. He could no more hear Penny's tiny voice than he could hear a flower grow.

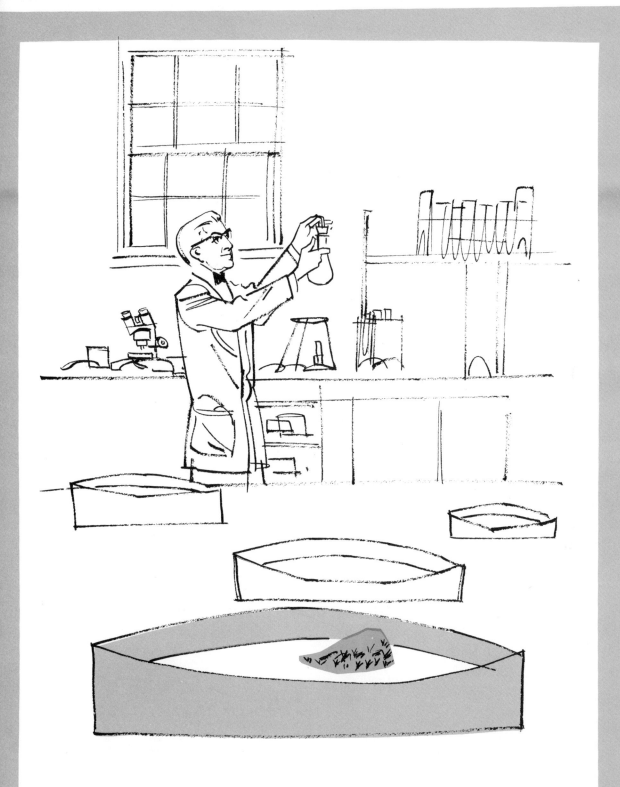

Penny's tribe all took a deep breath and shouted together: "DR. FLEMING! HERE'S SOME PENICILLIN!"

Dr. Fleming paused. Was that the wind whispering? The tribe took an enormous breath and screamed:

"DR. FLEMING! HERE'S SOME PENICILLIN!"

Dr. Fleming looked down at the dish. "My goodness," he said; "look at this interesting stuff. Maybe this will help kill those awful Strep germs."

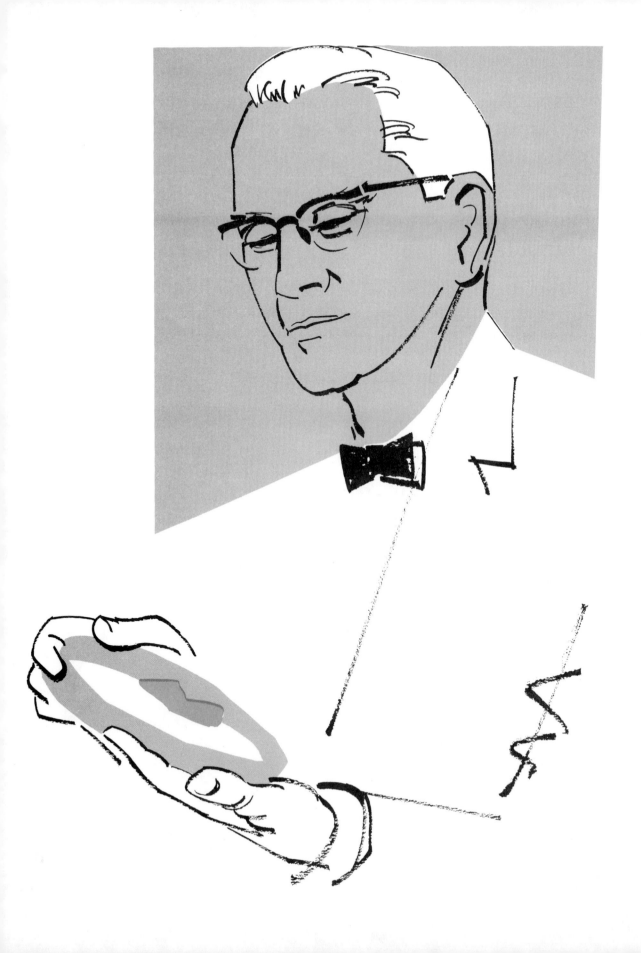

"Yes, yes!" the tribe said. "Let us at them!"

Dr. Fleming showed the penicillin to his friend, Dr. Florey, who injected it into the little boy. The penicillin swam into the boy's ear, shouting:

Chase those Strep!
Keep in step!
Out they go—
Fast! Not slow!
Use that pep!
Goodbye, Strep!

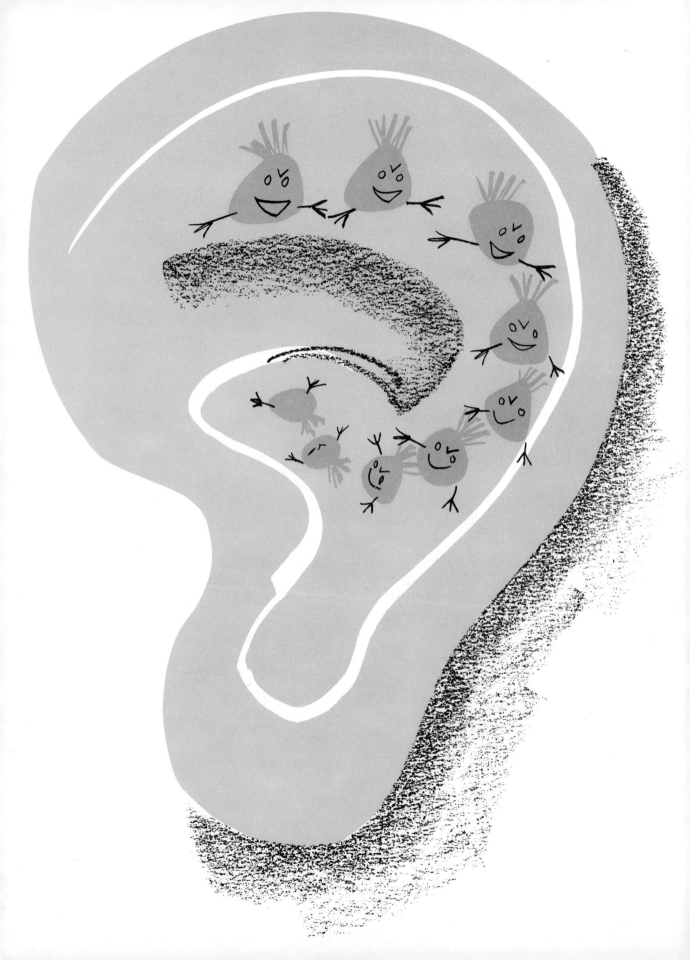

The Strep germs disappeared in the flood of liquid the penicillin family had oozed into the sore ear. By morning, the little boy's ear had lost most of its soreness, and Penny's snug home was ready for him again.

But a funny thing had happened. Penny no longer wanted to lie around napping.

"Now that we have Dr. Fleming and Dr. Florey to help, we can cure ears and throats all over the world," Penny told his tribe. "Let's go!"

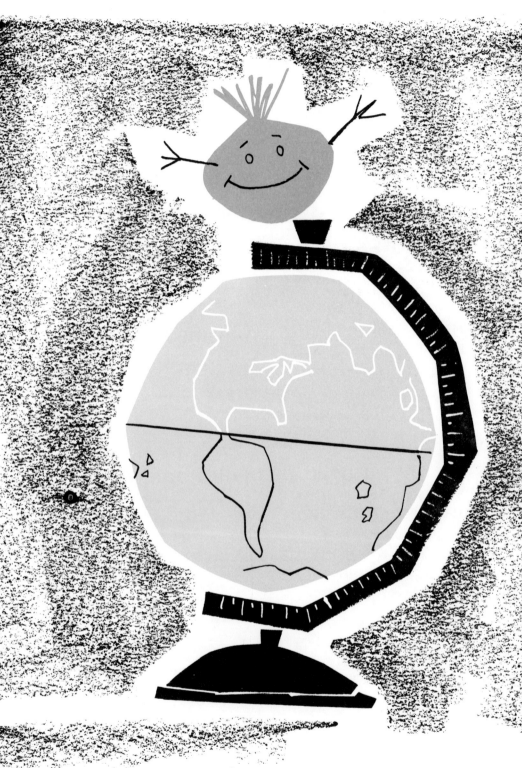

Dr. Florey taught doctors everywhere how to use penicillin. Before long, they found that Penny could get rid of those other bullies, the Staph and the Pneumos. From that day to this, Penny and his tribe have been busy curing boys and girls, and their fathers and mothers, too.

Next time you need penicillin, maybe you can pretend you hear the song the good germs made up that first exciting day:

Chase those Strep!

Keep in step!

Out they go—

Fast! Not slow!

Use that pep!

Goodbye, Strep!

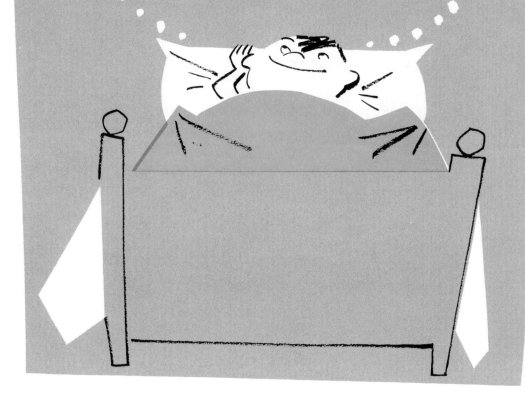

And, if you listen very carefully, you may hear the verse they added later:

> Those old Staph
> Make us laugh!
> Pneumos drop
> Plop! Last stop!
> Penicillin's
> Bad for villains!
> Bet they wish some other fellow
> Landed in that dish of jello!

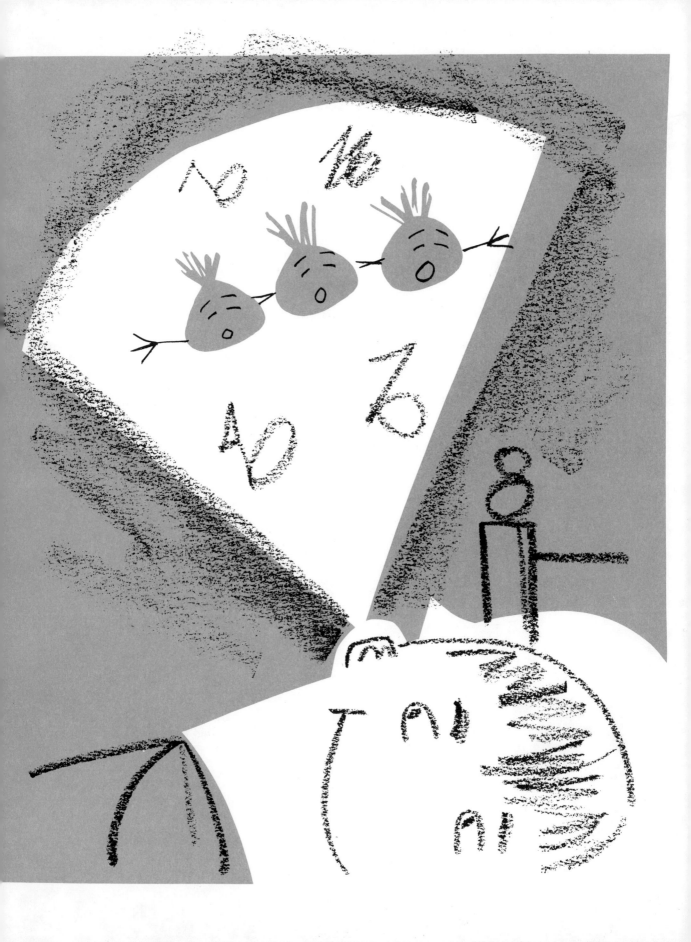

Information on the Discovery of Penicillin

In London, England, in 1928, spores (or seeds) of the mold *Penicillium notatum* happened to blow in through an open window in Dr. Alexander Fleming's pathology laboratory in St. Mary's Hospital. They alighted on an uncovered Petri dish containing agar, a nutrient material that looks like jello, on which staphylococci had been growing.

Dr. Fleming noticed that wherever the green mold, resembling the growth on stale bread or cheese, came in contact with the staph, the staph seemed to dissolve. He began to study this phenomenon and named the substance secreted by the mold penicillin. Dr. Fleming discovered that although penicillin was powerful in destroying certain germs, it did not harm the body tissues. He was unable to produce penicillin in stable form or large amounts, however, and for ten years little was done with it.

In 1938, at Oxford University, Dr. Howard Florey and Dr. E. B. Chain attempted to produce it in a usable form. By 1940 they had succeeded, but by then England was at war and no factories could be spared for the production of penicillin. Dr. Florey came to the United States in 1941. He persuaded the chief of the United States Department of Agriculture research laboratory to begin the production of penicillin. By late 1943 it was in fairly wide use in the Allied armies, and by 1945 enough was being produced by the American pharmaceutical industry to supply civilian needs as well.

Parents and teachers will be interested to know that, except for those relatively few people who are allergic to it, penicillin is one of the least toxic, or harmful, substances known. It is useful only against certain bacteria which cause boils, blood poisoning, scarlet fever, ear and throat infections, meningitis, and gas gangrene. It cures most venereal diseases. It is of absolutely no use against the common cold or against other diseases caused by viruses. It is not useful against those germs which generally cause diarrhea or kidney infections.

Because of the widespread use of penicillin, many strains of staphlococci have, unfortunately, become resistant to it so that not all infections caused by staphlococci can be cured by penicillin. Penicillin is, however, valuable in the treatment of most infections. It can be taken by mouth or by injection.

Important: Penicillin should not be used without medical supervision.

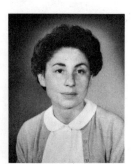

ABOUT THE AUTHOR

Sherrie S. Epstein lives with her husband Dr. Franklin H. Epstein, Associate Professor of Internal Medicine at Yale University, and three children in Hamden, Connecticut. Her previous writing experience has been along the lines of research and editing for the Government, for the New York University Press, and for an advertising agency. This is her first children's book.

Dr. Epstein told his children a version of this story to help explain to them why they needed penicillin for those recurrent ear infections. They enjoyed it and eagerly lapped up their good medicine. At this time, Mrs. Epstein was reviewing children's books in conjunction with the Connecticut Association for Mental Health and decided that this story was worth telling to all children.

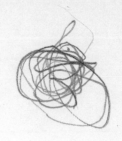
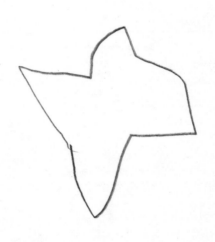